My Journey with the Devil's Disease

Lessons I Learned through My Lady's Struggle with Alzheimer's

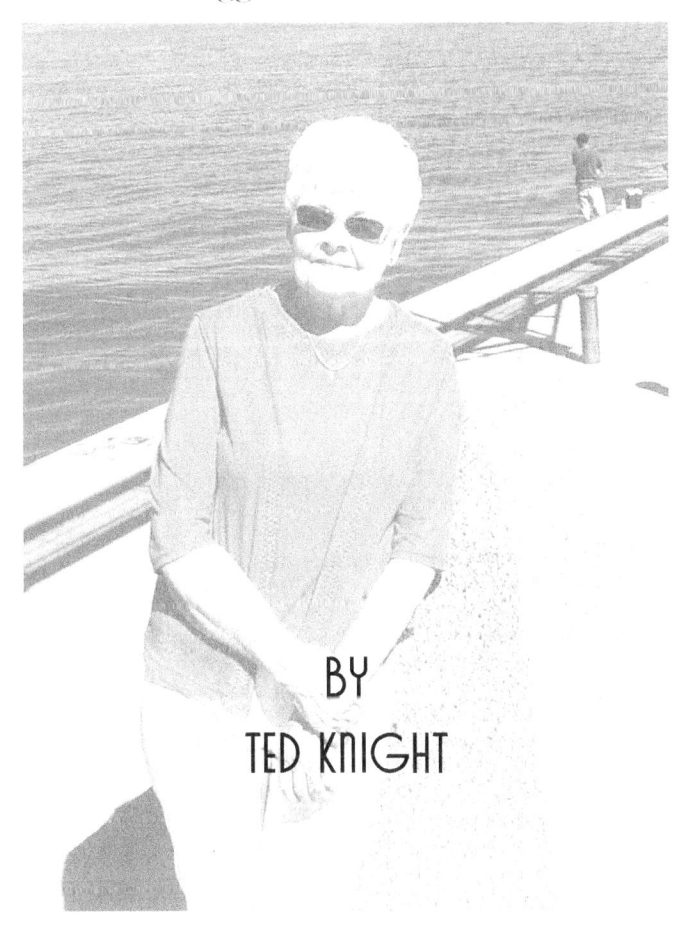

By
Ted Knight

My Journey with the Devil's Disease is copyright © 2023 by Ted Knight. All rights reserved.

Published in the United States of America by:
Cobb Publishing
704 E. Main St.
Charleston, AR 72933
Editor@CobbPublishing.com
www.CobbPublishing.com
479.747.8372

ISBN: 978-1-960858-17-7

Dedicated to

My Lady. The woman who cheered my life for our journey of 64 years and 96 days together. Even through the most difficult times, there is no one I would rather have been with than her, Barbara Jean Knight.

I await the time when I can join you again, together in heaven, praising God.

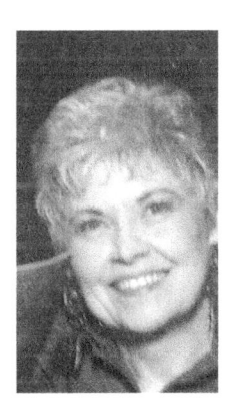

Foreword

In May 2019 I visited my parent's home because I had grown concerned about behaviors I had seen exhibited by my mother. When I asked my father if he had noticed the same things, he told me she had been diagnosed with Alzheimer's about twelve months earlier. Shortly thereafter Mom entered the room and I asked her to sit with me. I took her hand and said, "Dad tells me you have a problem. What's going on?"

With the combination of candor, honesty and humor that made communicating with my mother a delight, she said, "Well, son, I'm losing my mind."

At that moment, the journey with Alzheimer's that she and Dad had been on for twelve months became a reality for the rest of the family.

Mom was blessed with a remarkable set of life skills. Though her formal education was limited by today's standards, she possessed a keen intellect; an inordinate level of emotional intelligence; a significant ability to think critically; an uncommon gift for communication; and a genuine, faith-based love for people. Aside from her leaving us on this earth, the most challenging part of this journey for me was watching those God-given set of skills fade away.

The decision to make known publicly a significant life challenge is agonizing. The family struggled with whether or not Mom deserved privacy regarding her condition. We balanced that against the fact that her life had touched thousands of others, many of whom loved Mom dearly. Finally, on August 12, 2019, the family posted this letter to social media.

Friends and Loved Ones,

There are times when the choice to make public something about one's life is difficult. Over the past several months, our family has been faced with such a choice.

In May 2018, our wife, mother, and grandmother was diagnosed with Alzheimer's. God blessed her with a beautiful smile and a loving heart that has resulted in hundreds, if not thousands, of friendships over her lifetime. We have struggled with how and when to share this with all of you. We feel that the time has come to do so.

She still feels well and recognizes everyone, but her condition is beginning to affect her conversations and mannerisms. She can become confused when she is asked a lot of questions or is in stressful situations.

As a family, we are learning much about this disease and what we must do to support her and meet her needs. Arrangements have been made for assistance with cooking and housework. Of course, we are doing our best to make sure that she has the best medical care possible.

We've learned that it is best not to ask a person with this condition if they remember something or someone. If you see her, please greet her and visit with her as you always have. A gentle reminder of who you are might be needed and is appropriate and welcome. Use of the phone can be confusing to her, but she would absolutely love to hear from you by card, letter, or a personal visit.

While this circumstance will require some changes to the work that Ted and Barbara have done for the Lord over the past 60-plus years, they plan to continue those efforts as long they can. Ted will be sharing additional information with the churches and individuals who support that work.

Our family is cherishing today and leaving tomorrow with God. Barbara's lifetime of faith and optimism has taught us to live in the moment and not dwell on what the future holds. While we remain positive and rely upon God's blessings, we do ask for your prayers on her behalf as this journey continues. We also ask that you pray for our dad, father, and grandfather in his role as her primary caregiver.

With much love,

Ted, Marty, Kathy and Family

There were many who helped care for Mom over the 4.5 years that she dealt with this dreadful disease. While many of us provided assistance, the heaviest burden was carried by Dad. As I mentioned at Mom's memorial service, in their 64 years of marriage she never lived a day outside his home. My sister and I are eternally grateful for the commitment between our parents. The love that Dad has for Mom is demonstrated in every single word of this book. I love him for that.

Communicating through the written word is a gift that Dad inherited from his mother. Once Mom's condition was made public, Dad began using social media to share his thoughts about their journey. This book is a compilation of his thoughts. Each family's journey with dementia is unique. If you are on that path with a loved one there will be things in this book that resonate with you; other things may not. It is my hope and prayer that you find this book useful and inspiring.

Marty Knight

Barbara Jean Knight

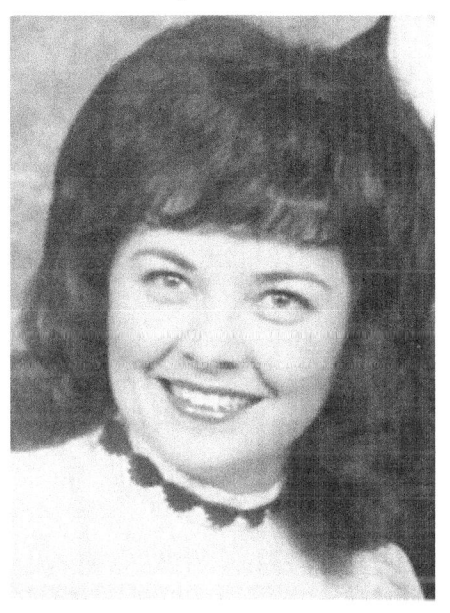

Barbara Knight was born at Caraway, Arkansas on September 17, 1941. Her family moved to Bay, Arkansas, when she was a small child and she lived there until 1958.

She was married to Ted Knight, also of Bay, Arkansas, when she was sixteen years of age. The two met when Ted was seven and Barbara was five. Following their wedding they moved to Michigan City, Indiana, intending to come back home to Bay after three months. They never returned to live there. She became a preacher's wife in 1959 and they lived together for 64 years and 96 days as husband and wife and Preacher and Preacher's wife for all of that time.

My Lady and I had grown up together, went to church together, school together, and worked in the fields together. Our families were very close. She came home with my sister one Sunday afternoon and that evening as we got in the car together to go to the evening assembly, I guess that I took her hand in mine, and since she didn't slap it away as we rode all the way to that evening assembly, I thought that she liked me. Not long after that we went to an after-church-service party with all the teens. We played a game called 'Spin the bottle' and when it pointed at her the two of us went on a walk down the road. On the way back, under a bright, beautiful moon I kissed her and I knew that she was mine. Neither of us ever dated anyone else and on July 24, 1958 we became man and wife at my parent's home at Herman Junction. It was the greatest day of my earthly life. I cannot describe how much we loved each other.

Barbara lived through some very difficult times during her 81 years of life, and was a conqueror over many things by the grace of God and a diligent spirit of her own. In 1974 their son, Marty (age 12) was diagnosed with the most rapidly spreading cancer known, with only two cases of it known before. Barbara was extremely exhaustive in her effort to not let this disease take her firstborn child. She, with her husband began immediately to find the best help that they could find, seeking advice and counsel rom Dr. John Ingle from Oklahoma City, OK, who discovered the cancer, Dr. William (Bill) Hodges from North Little Rock, Arkansas, who directed them to St. Jude's Hospital in Memphis, Tennessee. An entire book could be written about the excellent care afforded to Marty by St. Jude's hospital.

In 1995 Barbara was diagnosed with throat cancer by Dr. James Doug Stroud of Conway, Arkansas, who dedicated himself to seeing that she was given the most effective care that could be found for her. After receiving 25 Radiology treatments she recovered from that cancer.

In 1998 Barbara was diagnosed with breast cancer and had surgery by Dr. Charles Fielder of North Little Rock, Arkansas, and the battle to overcome began again and she was blessed to be victorious again.

The following consists of some things that I learned during the four years and six months that I served as her major caregiver. This is nothing like a deep study of things, just a day-to-day journey with the devils disease. We were told she could live up to 18 years with this disease. She lacked one day living 4 ½ years. So, those who lived with it for more years will have a lot more to say than this. If it is helpful to anyone I am thankful. Here is my final post:

If it is helpful to someone, I am thankful and give God the glory.

Ted Knight

A Journey With The Devil's Disease: ALZHEIMERS

I do not remember when I began making this journal as we moved along through this journey. It was probably about 3 years into the journey that I began keeping notes from a caregiver's view. She did really well for the first 2 ½ years and then it slowly became apparent the disease was really beginning to worsen. It was at that point I began writing these things primarily for myself at that time.

SOME THINGS I LEARNED AS A CAREGIVER WITH MY LADY

I am learning that the tone of one's voice when talking is as important or even more so, than what is said. Things seem so simple to me and I wonder why she does what she does or doesn't do what she should. I would lay her clothes out for her to wear that day, but when I saw her come out of the bedroom she would be dressed completely in different clothes. Therefore, my tone of voice may have been gruff at times and it shouldn't have been because she simply didn't understand. Use a soft and loving spirit as much as possible.

I am learning that a person with Alzheimer's can look directly at an object within twelve inches of their eyes and not see it. Or, see it in a different color, size, or shape. For instance, My Lady put on a pair of black shoes. Within five minutes I saw she had changed into a pair of white shoes. I asked her why she changed to white shoes and she very firmly said, "These are black shoes!"

I am learning that the loneliness of the caregiver of a person with Alzheimer's can be very hard to deal with. Caregiving is a difficult work and one that should not be done by just one person. Family and friends can make a huge difference in the life of one who is confined and caring for a loved one.

I am learning that a reasonable conversation comes briefly and goes away quickly at times. We may be having a rational conversation, and suddenly her response to something that is said is completely irrational. We would be talking about a trip that was coming up, and I would begin talking about it and her response would, "Are the kids coming this afternoon to help with putting up some pictures?"

I am learning that the need to control your temper and be kind is absolutely essential—even if it is so very difficult to do. When the afflicted person is unkind and loses his/her temper, the caregiver must not respond in that way. It is time to quietly and gently walk away, or it is time for a loving and gentle hug.

I am learning that someone who has never personally dealt with Alzheimer's or lived with it 24 hours a day, 7 seven days a week, is not qualified to give counsel or advice to the one who has. There may be helpful books or doctors who can help us deal with some of the emotions that Alzheimer's brings to the caregiver but living with it 24/7 is a challenge that only the one involved can understand. I have been blessed immensely by our family and I could not have dealt with this without their help. However dealing with it alone would be a load that few could bear.

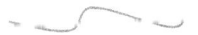

I have learned that others who have lived with Alzheimer's 24/7 are the best counselors. Experience is the best teacher, I have heard, and I believe it is true. I treasure some of the things I have been given by those who have prior experience in caregiving, although even then it is something to bear alone to really grasp. Every case is different and what was effective in one instance may not be best at all in another case.

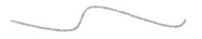

I am learning that the patient can see other people and hear their voices when they are not there. These people often tell the Alzheimer's patient to do things and say things that obviously are not true except to the patient. "They" have become a full time resident of our house although they are not there.

I am reaffirming my belief that it is ok and even good to be able to cry. Cheeks bathed in tears are not signs of weakness and fear or a lack of faith, but avenues of relief from pain. I say, "Cry often. Whatever the need, to relieve pain or express joy and happiness, just go ahead and cry."

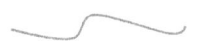

I am learning the importance of ignoring words and actions, and after a few seconds moving on to something else. Deflection is a very good and important tool to use every day. When you are surprised when the patient says, "I think that it is snowing, and in reality it is 90 degrees outside, just move on to something else without beginning an argument.

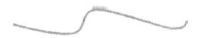

I am learning to be grateful for friends who 'prop us up on the leaning side.' May God bless you every one. A phone call, a brief visit, or even a card can be very encouraging. Please do not think that you will be imposing with a phone call or visit. It will be OK to call and ask if it is OK to come for a visit. You are needed for that. I am feeling the importance of prayer, and it is yours that we seek today.

AND THE JOURNEY CONTINUES... We love you, Roy and Dale.

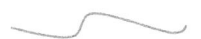

I have learned that the people My Lady is with has a great bearing on how she feels even several hours later. My daughter and her husband recently went with us on a trip that was a little more than 48 hours long, and we drove almost 1000 miles. The trip was very pleasant and My Lady had no problems staying in a hotel two nights and all the travel. But, there are other times when she has been with someone for a much shorter time and became very nervous and it took several hours for her to become comfortable again. Be careful and pleasant in your communication with an Alzheimer's patient and don't go over your problems with them, lest they become overly concerned about your problems and their problems become worse.

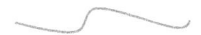

I have learned the importance of allowing My Lady to do what she can do, even if she makes a mess of something and I have to do it over. I have been too impatient and wanted her to just sit down and let me fold the clothes, load the dishwasher, etc., like I wanted them done. Now, she helps with those things and she feels like she is helping even if I have to slip around and do something over. It is very important that she feels some value and believes that there are some things that she can do.

I have learned it is really good for people to realize she isn't the 'bubbling over with personality Barbara' that she has always been, and to realize that when she talks to them about chopping or picking cotton the day before, just get in the cotton patch for a moment with her and she will be happy.

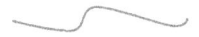

I have learned it is very easy to scare her and that this should not be done. Words can scare her and images can scare her, even if they are not real. If I respond to something from her or even on TV, my response by word or deed may scare her. There must be great care in trying to joke with an Alzheimer's patient because things that may have been funny to her in the past are not funny now.

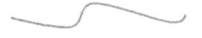

I have learned that both of us are going through a tough transition in our life. It is not of her doing and she must not be held accountable for it. It is the disease that very often speaks and acts—and not the My Lady that I have had for so many decades.

I have learned that we can still laugh at all kinds of things. We remember in our past things that we laugh at and enjoy remembering. I try to make her laugh as much as possible because laughter may indeed be "The Best Medicine." Even when we cry together, when the crying is over we find reason to laugh at ourselves.

I have learned that some people seem to think she is contagious and they don't need to be around us. We need company. We need fellowship. We don't need to be ignored as though something is really wrong with us, even though something is wrong with us and your fellowship with us might be good medicine for both of us.

I have learned that TV can be very dangerous for her if it isn't something along "Andy Griffith" lines. If you know of a good movie that we might watch, let us know and that would be good for both of us. The NEWS is definitely a "NO-NO."

I have learned that what she eagerly ate for lunch yesterday is a horrible suggestion for lunch today. When I remind her how much she liked it, she tells me that it made her really, really sick and not to offer that again. Two days later she ate it just fine. That is Alzheimer's at work.

I have learned to include her in everything possible just as if there is nothing wrong. She doesn't need to be made to believe that something is drastically wrong with her and that she cannot participate.

I have learned to be as loving and tender as I possibly can when she tells me that she knows what she has and where it is taking her. This is the hardest thing that I have to deal with, because I want to tell her that she is wrong but I know that she isn't. She is far too smart medically to try to tell her everything is alright. She fully knows at times, when she is mentally alert, what the problem is and where it is taking her.

AND THE JOURNEY CONTINUES...

I have learned that 'little things' become 'BIG' things to an Alzheimer's patient. And, some very important things are not important at all to that patient. It is very difficult to know the difference but when the caregiver discovers it and makes adjustments it can be very important. Listening to the patient can help the caregiver immensely.

I have learned that when the time comes, and is right, have some fun. Laugh and giggle about things especially things that the patient thinks are funny. Make these sessions last as long as possible. The memories will be precious jewels in the future.

I have learned to cherish those moments when she seems almost as normal as she has ever been. It may be five minutes, or more, or less, but make them as long as they can be before they are lost again.

I have learned that when she sees things and people that are not there, don't argue about them, just see those things and people in your own mind and go along. Remember, those things and people are real to her and they will pass sooner or later.

I have learned that there are things of the past that she seems to remember clearly and probably will forever. For instance, she was a part of a group of about 15 girls in school that has continued their friendship for all of these years. She still talks to some of them on the phone. You would not believe how many times "the girls" have told her to do things and say things that are just out of the blue sky. "The girls" are so very important to her and I hope that memory will last as long as she does.

I have learned and continue to learn that schedules, eating, sleeping, etc. are out the window. She may eat a wonderful lunch and two hours later ask when we are having lunch. She may wake up at 4 o'clock AM and think she is late getting in the shower. I can usually talk her out of that, but not always. Alzheimer's requires some adjusting when it comes to schedules. It is almost like raising a toddler again.

I have learned that when she is crying for no apparent reason, just stay quietly nearby and let her cry. Soon, she will be ok. But I have learned that the more I talk and try to reason with her, the crying just goes on and on. After all, don't we all want to just curl up and have a good cry occasionally?

I have learned that Alzheimer's is the culprit, not My Lady. She may do things that are totally out of character for her. It is NOT her! It is Alzheimer's and she has no more control over it than I do. Want to place blame somewhere? Put it where it belongs, on Satan and his partner Alzheimer's, and not the patient.

I have learned that I am not a real good beautician, hair stylist, or make-up artist, but I sure do have a great looking Lady to practice on. She has been beautiful all of her life, and I just love it when she is all made up.

I have learned that sleep is a very real friend, especially if you have good dreams. Sometimes the confusion begins as soon as our feet hit the floor and continues until we get in the bed that night. A full night of sleep is seldom enjoyed. It is an awful intrusion into what could have been a very good day.

I have learned that it is OK to be angry, but that anger must be properly directed. I really get angry sometimes, not at her but at that monster that lives in her head and is constantly eating away at her brain and cannot be stopped. I hate that monster because of what it is robbing me of...My Lady!

I have learned that I have not appreciated what My Lady has done for 63 years and 61 days in our home. Now that I am doing so much of what she has done, I cannot imagine why I was so blind to her efforts. Only God knows how hard she worked but made it look easy for us to have a home like we have enjoyed.

I have learned that when you think you cannot take another step, Jesus will give you another step and one step at a time is all that we can take to continue the journey. And if you try to walk this journey without God and Jesus, you will not make it with anything left of yourself.

AND THE JOURNEY CONTINUES...

I have learned that most of the caregiver's problems stem from exhaustion. Therefore some provision for rest must be made or the task becomes much more difficult. There have been times when I have thought that I could not take another step but

I did. So, find a time to get some rest, you are going to need it.

I have learned over and over again that God is by far the most important part of the triangle involving My Lady the Alzheimer's patient, Me the Care Giver, and God. Time must be made for reading, study, and prayer. Without that, the battle will be lost for both parties.

I have learned that My Lady often thinks I am angry just by the response to something that she did that surprised and sometimes shocked me. That will happen over and over. In many cases the caregiver expects more than the patient can give, and it is very frustrating. For instance, you may think that when she is in the shower she will remember everything involved. But be ready for the patient to want to use shampoo for soap and vice versa. The patient will want to get out of the shower while still dripping wet and you have to help them dry off. So, careful attention needs to be given to every response.

I have learned over and over that my mouth needs to be kept shut sometimes, and after so long of having it open nearly all the time whether it needed to be or not, that is quite a challenge. Quietness for the Alzheimer's patient can be a good thing.

I have learned to be very careful in teasing her because what has been teasing in the past and was acceptable, may not be considered teasing at all anymore.

I have learned that the caregiver must be extra alert when it comes medicine-taking time. The correct medicine, the correct dosage, the correct times, and making sure that the medicine is taken and not poured out, all must be carefully attended to. Sometimes the patient my just pour it all out before the caregiver can stop it, but there is always another dose that can be administered. Don't make a mess out of the medicine-taking time.

I have learned that it is very important to be alert all of the time, even during the night, because you never know when she will get into something that she shouldn't or even go somewhere outside. It happens in the blinking of the eye. She may start to use deodorant for tooth paste and you see it out of the corner of your eye and jump to stop it. Or, she may wander off to Marty and Lisa's next door, but doesn't know which house they are in. So, being alert at all times is important.

I have learned to dislike it when she does something that in other circumstances might be considered funny, but it isn't funny to her or to me, and I don't want her to be laughed at by me or anyone else. My anger is on a light trigger when it comes to someone laughing at her. Alzheimer's isn't funny.

AND THE JOURNEY CONTINUES...

I have learned that it is very important that she eat properly. She has never been a big eater. She can eat a good meal at breakfast time and not be hungry until the next big breakfast. She has always been that way, but now she may want to eat five times a day with a few snacks in between. And the doctor says, "That's good, let her eat." It may be good for the doctor, but he doesn't have to have the food ready when she gets hungry.

I have learned to do everything that I can to avoid thinking about tomorrow and to live in the moment and be as content as I can. If tomorrow comes we will deal with it and if tomorrow doesn't come it will be wonderful to be at rest or at home with God.

I have learned to grab hold of the peace that comes from knowing that the Godhead, God, Jesus, and the Holy Spirit, are present with us at all times. We talk almost every night about God, Jesus, and the Holy Spirit being in our bedroom with us. Yes, we know that Satan is there as well but he can do nothing that the other three cannot handle.

I have learned that there is great value in pictures to her. My Lady's younger sister, Lin Rahrle has come to visit many times and spent most of her time hanging pictures for us. My lady loves those pictures and goes over and over them every day, looking at them as though it was the first time she has seen them. The same thing is true with greeting cards. She reads them over and over again as though she has never seen them before. Say, you might invest 59 cents postage and a 50 cent card at Dollar Tree and bring some light to My Lady.

I have learned that it is futile to try to explain something to an Alzheimer's patient. When they do something wrong it is useless to try to explain that it's wrong because to them it is not wrong. The argument that such efforts bring proves to be detrimental to both the caregiver and the patient.

I have learned to try not to be surprised with far-fetched ideas that an Alzheimer's patient may have. It may be from Mars, but so be it. Just move with it back to Mars where it came from and love your loved one. My Lady has come up with some things that are far-out and then when she realizes what she had said, we both have a good laugh together.

I have learned that adjusting over and over again is the rule of living with Alzheimer's. I believe that it will continue as long as the disease remains. Food tastes change, bedtime and getting up times change. The time for a shower changes and often she will say she just got out of the shower when she hasn't. So adjusting is absolutely necessary. Refusing to adjust leads to chaos and confusion for the patient as well as the caregiver.

I have learned that there are many things money will not buy—and a cure for Alzheimer's at this time is one of them. Rumors abound about the cure for Alzheimer's has been found and people share those things with me, but they simply are not true. Money will not buy a cure, but it may assist the researchers in someday discovering the cure. If I owned Fort Knox I would find there is no cure for Alzheimer's there. And, by the way, I don't own Fort Knox.

I have learned that Alzheimer's does not leave two people in a fifty/fifty situation. There is no giving and taking. Caring for an Alzheimer's patient requires almost 100% of the caregiver's time and effort while the patient is oblivious to what is going on. The caregiver does the giving and hopes that the patient will do the getting.

AND THE JOURNEY CONTINUES...

I have learned that sights and sounds in the night are of concern to her. Every house I have ever known has had some squeak or pop during the night and they were never a concern to her before. Now the slightest sound tells her that someone is in the house or trying to get in the house. The biggest culprit is the icemaker in the refrigerator. It grunts and groans like some drunk and really upsets her until I explain what it is. The shadow of the fan blades on the ceiling scare her almost every day until I explain to her what they are.

I have learned that an Alzheimer's patient should be treated with the greatest respect. Who they are with Alzheimer's and who they were before are two entirely different people. But, the one that was, is still in the one that is, somewhere, and deserves the same respect if not greater than before. I firmly believe that what the patient once was and what they knew is hidden away somewhere and cannot get out. I realize that there comes a time when the disease has become more aggressive and become more acute, they may not be aware of anything that goes on.

I have learned that when an Alzheimer's patient is awake, they seldom stop moving. There is something that they feel needs to be changed in some way, hidden away for some reason, or completely disposed of. So, don't be surprised at what you find in the refrigerator, bathroom, shower, or commode that should not be there. The things that are yours may show up sometime in the strangest place and you will know who put them there and you will never know *why* they did it. (There are two rings, one of mine and one of hers that look a lot alike, that are missing and have been for months.)

I have learned that My Lady Alzheimer's patient should not have her personal needs neglected simply because she is an Alzheimer's patient. So, we get up, get her in the shower, I lay her clothes out as I have done for years, we do her hair and makeup, and get her ready for the day. I want her to look as beautiful as I can for as long as we can. She deserves it even if I have to hire someone to help us get it done. My Lady has been a Lady of dignity and grace and she will receive that kind of attention as long as I live to provide it for her.

I have learned that I just thought I had been tired before, but now I know I had only touched the hem of the garment. A caregiver must be ready almost 24 hours a day because of the up and downs that the patient has. And, I look at her and know that inside she is far more tired than me because she knows to some degree what is happening.

I have learned and continue to learn that a one-way conversation is not very enjoyable. I make a comment and the response often is completely off the wall not even close to the remark that I made. That happens so often and it is so frustrating. What do we do in that situation? Drop your head a bit to keep from showing your frustration and disappointment and reach over and take her hand and say, "I love you," and move on in a little bit with something that she may be familiar with. Then, when you get the chance, cry your heart out and feel better.

I have learned and continue to learn that I need to learn as much as I can about life with Alzheimer's as we move along. I must not overlook anything that might be helpful down the road. I know that the disease is going to progress and there will be new lessons to learn and that I will need help. Be aware!

AND THE JOURNEY CONTINUES...

I have learned that when I learn something that I want to share with you, I need to write it down right then or a short time later what I learned didn't stay learned very long. The caregiver's brain is challenged every day to learn and remember Alzheimer's lessons. Caregiving is a fulltime job with other things taking a back seat a lot of the time.

I have learned that it is hard to know which is worse...the constant talking and going from one to another thing that makes no sense at all and I know nothing about, or the deafening silence when she doesn't talk at all. It is like the very active child who makes a lot of noise or the child who is almost entirely silent.

I have learned to lean on people like Dale Smith and others who have been on this journey far longer than we have and can offer much help to all who struggle with Alzheimer's. Playing it alone can be disastrous. Find someone who loves you and take them along on the journey. If you have someone to 'prop you up on the leaning side,' that person is worth more than a lot of advice from people who mean well but don't know what they are talking about.

I have learned that as difficult as it is for me to admit it, I need help. When I said, "I do for better or worse, for richer or for poorer," I meant it and I was determined to take care of her in every situation in life. Now, there is a load that I cannot carry without God, family, and friends to help me. I sat in the Doctor's office recently and could not believe that I was telling him that I needed him, even though he has been our family doctor for 46 years. I have often preached and written that "We need each other," and I know it now better than I did before.

I have learned that some people are not very conscious of what they say to and in front of an Alzheimer's patient. Although we know that the patient has Alzheimer's and we think they cannot understand us, we are very wrong. They understand much more of what we say than we think they do and the results are often very painful to both patient and caregiver who is left to try to explain that no hurt was intended.

I have learned, and this may be a bit blunt...But, some who were friends before this disease came, are not very friendly and evidently were not the friends we thought they were. There is never or very, very seldom a visit, phone call, card, or anything else that they could do to share our burden. Blunt, but painfully true.

I have learned the inestimable value of every minute that I get to spend with her. I know that sometimes it is very, very difficult to spend hours on end with her and that my children and many of you tell me I must get away and take care of myself. But, I know that every minute that I am away from her is a minute I can never regain. I know that when I am away from her in body, I am with her in mind, so it is not possible to really get away. So, I must get every minute with her that I can and still maintain my own mental and physical state. So, I say to other loved ones, "Don't let too many minutes pass without being with that loved one because the number of minutes is passing by rapidly."

I have learned that it is OK to be scared. I am not John Wayne or Clint Eastwood. I am not David but I know I am facing a Goliath. Sometimes I find myself mentally and physically just scared half to death but God picks me up and helps me to go again.

AND THE JOURNEY CONTINUES...

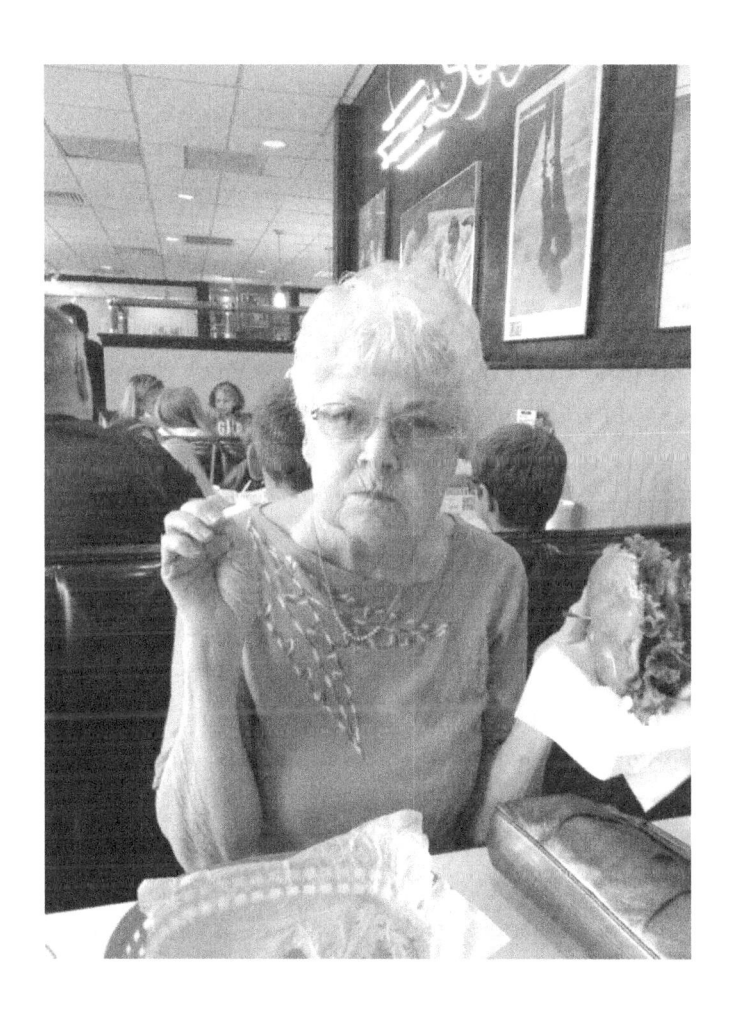

I have learned that time means nothing to an Alzheimer's patient because they cannot tell time. And when I ask her for five minutes to get something done, she comes two minutes later and wants to help me. I must move along in life with a fraction of the time that I did have to get my work done. She doesn't mean to, but she demands time that I need for myself and for my work.

I have learned to accept that my expectations may not become reality. I keep telling myself that when we get up in the morning all of this will have been taken away and we will return to normal, but I know that isn't going to happen unless God intervenes.

I have learned that when she needs to cry, I need to just hold her and let her cry. And, that usually results in both of us crying and that's when the only place to go is to God. I believe that God created tears as a means of relief when our hearts are in pain. That is when God sees us and hears us with our cheeks bathed in tears. Normally the relief that we feel when the crying is over is almost worth it. A great load has been lifted off of us.

Today I have learned that today I can count my blessings because...

- Today I still have her and she still knows me and we can still communicate well... I'll take it.
- Today I still have her and she has a good appetite and eats real well... I'll take it.
- Today I still have her and her medications still seem to work well... I'll take it.
- Today I still have her and she is as beautiful as ever... I'll take it.
- Today I still have her and so many, many, people still love her dearly... I'll take it.
- Today I still have her and when I forget the words to a song, she reminds me... I'll take it.
- Today I still have her and she can still take care of almost all of her personal needs... I'll take it.
- Today I still have her and she still loves her lipstick... I'll take it.
- Today I still have her and she still loves to assemble with the church and listen to me preach... I'll take it.
- Today I still have her and she is still a great example to our children, grandchildren,

great-grandchildren, and thousands of friends... I'll take it.
- Today I still have her and we will lay down to take a nap and five minutes later she will say, "I had a good nap." I will say, "You scoundrel, you didn't even take a nap" and ... I'll take it.
- Today I still have her and she will ask, "Is today church day?" ten times and I will tell her "No." and ... I'll take it.
- Today I still have her and she has no doctor appointment and is in good physical health and... I'll take it.
- Today I still have her and she will wake me up in the middle of the night saying, "Somebody's in this house," and I will catch her and say, "There's no one here but you and me," and she'll be happy with it and... I'll take it.
- Today I still have her and she will get me so frustrated and yes angry, but I will grit my teeth and get over it and... I'll take it.
-

I have learned that even small crowds and lots of noise really makes things difficult for My Lady. Why shouldn't it? Crowds and noise especially at sporting events bother me, so why shouldn't it bother someone with Alzheimer's? They become afraid and so these gatherings need to be avoided.

I have learned Alzheimer's is winning the battle over us mentally and physically. We cannot stop it and we certainly cannot dismiss it as though it isn't there. But its victory over us in those areas will mean victory FOR us spiritually and eternally. And that makes us Winners!

I have learned that one of the most difficult things to do with an Alzheimer's patient is to get them to sit down. My Lady just walks and walks looking for something that she never finds until I can sit down with her. It is hard to get her to sit down to eat a meal. For some reason she wants to stand and be active.

I have learned that the caregiver needs a good dose of extra education in the Fruit of the Spirit: "Love, joy, peace, longsuffering, gentleness, goodness, faith, meekness and temperance." These qualities all in abundance are needed with an Alzheimer's patient.

I have learned that what I learn today must be learned in a different way tomorrow because life has changed since yesterday. No two days are the same. Needs and desires change from day to day. Caregiving demands constantly changing.

I have learned that things come into her mind without any foundation for them at all. For instance, this morning she woke up feeling fine but in just minutes she became very upset because she realized that today was the day that she would die. She even saw herself in her casket. Be prepared for some very heart-breaking things.

I have learned that every day she becomes more conscious of what is happening to her and it is very painful to her. The days of not knowing what the problem is, is over. One of her closest and dearest friends of more than 56 years passed away after a long battle with this disease. We would go and see her and when we left she would cry and say, "I don't want to be like Peggy." That is exactly where she is headed unless the Lord would be merciful to her and change that destiny. (It was changed because Peggy lived more than twice the number of years than My Lady).

I have learned that sometimes the difference between being angry at the disease and being angry at her is very small. I must work diligently every day to remember, "It isn't her, it is Alzheimer's." Almost every day there is something that provokes anger of some sort and I emphasize to her and to myself over and over again, "This isn't you, this isn't you, it is your illness."

I have learned that it is very difficult to explain things to her. She said, "I have to live a different life now." I asked what she meant and she told me exactly that because of Alzheimer's she cannot live like me, our family, and others. She was correct and what do I say? She told me, "It's over." I again asked what she meant and she told me that her life is over and today she will die. How do you explain something to somebody who already knows what the explanation is... that we are all going to die but we do not know when? She knows that but in her mind for that moment, it is today.

AND THE JOURNEY CONTINUES...

I have learned that it is very hard to get her to eat when eating is the last thing she wants to do. Do you remember how difficult it was to get your child to eat? To get a sick adult to eat against his or her will is far more challenging. She does not get hungry and gets very aggravated when we try to insist that she eat. (Thirty minutes later she is starving.)

I have learned that one of the good stress relievers is to get out of the house and take a walk if possible or get in the car and take a drive. A stop at Andy's Frozen Custard place is a good idea or some other favorite place for a refreshment time. Four walls can get closed in pretty quick at times. I just have to ignore that those turtle sundaes are putting pounds on me too.

I have learned that smiles can turn to tears in a very, very short time and it is challenging for the caregiver to make that change. The caregiver's response can be one of frustration or even anger in such cases. The patient and the caregiver both are on an emotional roller coaster.

I have learned that the mental and physical health of the caregiver is of supreme importance to continue to provide care for the Alzheimer's patient. It is a tough road to travel, but it can be done if proper care is given to both the caregiver and patient.

I have learned that being a caregiver for an Alzheimer's patient is not a one-person task. Remember the saying, "It takes a village"? That is certainly the case in providing proper care for a loved one in this condition.

I have learned that holidays, especially ones like Thanksgiving and Christmas are quite painful for both the patient and caregiver. My patient is still conscious of things enough to know what holiday it is, but it is not the enjoyable time that it once was. Both of us hear of others having a great time and we are very limited in what we can do, so we try to enjoy as much as we can under the circumstances.

I have learned that I would love to have one more day with My Lady of five years ago or even 63 years and 135 days ago on our wedding day. She was so beautiful and so much a Lady and she continues to be that same way today. Oh, for one day with her before Alzheimer's came.

I have learned that Alzheimer's is a devil, eating away at the brain one small bit at a time until a person is totally helpless. It isn't a huge move that came one day but it is week, month, year, or even day of small moves that slowly diminishes the patient's ability to function.

I have learned that it is difficult to maintain a spirit of hope when the patient is slipping away and there is no stopping it. The challenge to give up and lose all hope constantly rears its ugly head and reminds us of the struggle we are fighting. There must be a heart full of prayer at all times.

I have learned that I need to go back and read again some of the things that I have already written and see that I have fallen far short of some of those things and that I need to listen to myself more often. It is easy to forget when dealing with an emotional tornado.

I have learned that so many, many, people have suffered a greater loss than we have and that prompts me to count my blessings and move on. When we are involved with our own problems we often forget that others are fighting their own battles as well.

AND THE JOURNEY CONTINUES...

I have learned that when patience is weak and anger is strong and in a conflict with an Alzheimer's patient and a caregiver, both lose and nobody wins. It is up to the caregiver to see that those times are as infrequent as possible and resolution reached quickly.

I have learned that those moments when everything seems normal must be tucked away and the memory cherished because those moments will melt away quickly. I love it when she lays with her head on my shoulder and we talk for a few minutes and everything is well until she slips away again.

I have learned the folly of trying to "explain" something to an Alzheimer's patient who will remember that explanation for two or three minutes and that which needed explaining will return. When the memory is so short there is need for repeating maybe several times within a short time. It may be tiresome and boring to the caregiver but it is needed for the patient.

I have learned that it would be a lie for me to say I have never been so angry I could hardly function and sought escape for a few moments. Frustration mounts as things continue until my teeth are clenched so that my entire head hurts. Those are times when crying out to God is the only recourse that one seems to have.

I have learned that it is alright to cry out, "WHY?" In fact I doubt that anyone has gone through life with Alzheimer's without crying out "WHY?" "WHY" such an intelligent, beautiful, loving person as this should be stricken with such a horrible disease? Sometimes the only answer is stark silence until we can grasp our focus and bring it under control until we let God answer. And answer He will if we will listen closely.

I have learned that long ago times of pain and sorrow which she thought were long ago forgotten, have reared their ugly heads now and are causing the same pain and sorrow as long ago. Three episodes of cancer and countless other times of real hard periods of illnesses have come back like they occurred yesterday to her. That is why it is important to have a good doctor who works with Alzheimer's patients to help them through these times. Oh, how I wish that I could remove these things forever from her memory but I doubt that it can ever be done. We have a very fine geriatric psychiatrist who has helped and we highly recommend this treatment.

I have learned that unexplainable spells of anger can cause an Alzheimer's patient to be an almost unrecognizable person from the one we have known for years. Offering to pray is one very good way to handle such a time, but if that is rejected, leaving the scene as quickly as possible without damage to her mental capacity is the best way to handle such a problem.

I have learned and re-learn daily to enjoy the sweet moments as often as they come and that is really often. This morning she said she was ready to get up, shower and get dressed. I told her she would have to get out of bed to do that. "Oh," she said and looked at me as though she was asking, "Why do I have to get out of bed to do that?" I love those times when we can laugh and joke and have fun.

AND THE JOURNEY CONTINUES...

I have learned that it is really important to enjoy life to the fullest when you can because that blessing may be changed drastically in a moment. No one intends to lose their ability to function fully and stay well but it can happen in the twinkling of an eye and you will be challenged in ways that you had never even considered before.

I have learned that some people are not as sensitive as they should be when laughing at something that is not normal. The Alzheimer's patient will wonder what they have done because to them it is normal to say or do the things that they say and do. All people should be doubly sensitive about laughing in the presence of an Alzheimer's patient. Honestly, I as the spouse and caregiver can be irritated when someone laughs at something that is not funny coming from someone who is sick with a horrible disease.

I have learned that stubbornness and anger accompany Alzheimer's. It is much better to show the patient how and why something should be done than to demand of them something that they have never liked and now it is even more distasteful to them. Showing rather than just telling is a much better plan. And again deflection is a good tool under such circumstances.

I have learned that it is advisable to talk to an Alzheimer's patient about their condition occasionally. For instance, tonight, Jan. 2, 2022, I got up on her side of the bed and told her, "I know that it isn't you when you become angry and stubborn, it is the medical problem that we are dealing with. I know that at times you do or say things that you didn't do before. So, we are going to live with it and it is going to be OK with me and the kids." It is amazing how much good that seemed to do for her. (I do not call it Alzheimer's to her because she despises the word Alzheimer's.)

I have learned that the changes that take place between the times we close our eyes at night and open them in the morning are many and at times shocking. That is how quickly the mental abilities are digressing. There is no 24 hour period that doesn't involve a small bit of change.

I have learned that the thought of just giving up sometimes looms large in the mind of a caregiver. When we know that there isn't going to be improvement but digression, it is hard to maintain a spirit of hope for the future. It passes quickly and we press on with trust in God and the assistance of family and friends.

I have learned to be appreciative of even the very small things that others do to give me an opportunity to have a little time to do my work or just walk up and down the street on a bright sunny day. A small bit of time for me to go to the post office or the bank is a very good contribution. Don't neglect to be aware that you may do a world of good by giving a few minutes of your time to assist someone.

AND THE JOURNEY CONTINUES...

I have learned that one of the most difficult things to deal with in an Alzheimer's patient is stubbornness. It is very challenging to get one to change their mind about a matter even if it is very important that they do so. It takes time and a gentle approach to turn a stubborn streak around.

———⌒———

I have learned that learning never stops with Alzheimer's disease. Every day something new arises and a caregiver must learn something new.

———⌒———

I have learned that the activating of the brain of the Alzheimer's patient is like the waves of the sea. When one comes in very high, shining in the sun, her mind is almost normal and for a brief time we have a conversation like we always did. But, the beautiful wave crashes and her mind with it and it is back to not being able to converse very well at all. But, I love those beautiful high waves that bristle in the sun.

———⌒———

I have learned that precious moments come and I love to store them away. She stood directly in front of a picture of her mother hanging on our wall. Her Mom has been gone for 69 years but My Lady still speaks of her nearly every day. As she stood there, suddenly she put her hand up to her mouth and kissed it and then reached out and planted that kiss on her mother's face. A more precious moment I haven't seen in a long, long time.

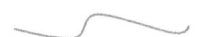

I have learned of the agony that comes with looking her straight in the eye and my seeing a beautiful, stunning, bright Lady who is pleading with me to let her come out and join me in the life that we have had for so long and I am frozen in the place where I can do nothing but love her and hold her and pray together.

I have learned that there needs to be, and I do not know where it is yet, a definitive line between not knowing something or a fit of anger and just plain meanness. I hate to make this statement but in the case of burst of anger one must learn to walk away—and it may not be a short walk, but one that will give the caregiver time to regain composure and settle down while the patient does too.

AND THE JOURNEY CONTINUES...

I have learned that trying to take the next step is very, very discouraging when you hardly know how to handle the present step. It is best to deal with the present moment and stop until the next moment comes. It is not 'one day at a time' but one moment at a time.

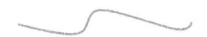

I have learned that a caregiver who is not a family member may sometimes do a more effective job than a family member. I have seen that when we are blessed with a helper from time to time. The ladies from hospice care were outstanding at getting her to do things that I could not do. Giving her a shower, which was sometimes a battle ground, was a simple thing for the hospice caregiver to do.

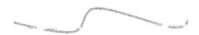

I have learned that the guilt that is felt when a wrong decision has been made can be the greatest pain that one can feel. It is very wise to consult others when a major decision is being considered. Is it time to call for hospice to come help? Has she reached the point when a hospital bed and other equipment need to be brought in? Tough decisions can be really draining and other family members should be consulted for relief for the caregiver.

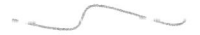

I have learned the heartache that comes from waking our son or daughter in the wee hours of the night is very heavy. Our son lives literally feet from us and our daughter lives just minutes away. Both they and their spouses are ready instantly to come help me when I call, but it is hard to wake them out of a deep sleep to come help me when I need them.

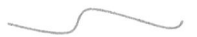

I have learned that she has almost lost the desire for affection and even to some degree a touch and, or an attempt to hold her provokes feelings of fear and what she perceives to be aggression on my part. She becomes afraid quickly. I miss so much the warmth and feelings of love and holding her in my arms. I miss the real her so very much.

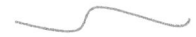

I have learned to be open to dealing with things that I never considered being a part of my life. But, I strive daily to be able to do those things without complaint for My Lady's sake. After all I may not have recognized it earlier, but how many times has she dealt with similar things for me? And, I know that if conditions were reversed she would be with me every minute that she could.

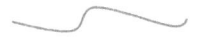

I have learned that I just thought that I loved her in the past I guess, because it seems that another whole batch of love has come from somewhere, God the Father, and I love her more each passing day. Not everything is easy and pleasant but with love everything is possible. Where love is not present nothing works out, but where love is present everything will work out fine.

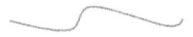

I have learned the awfulness of not having a reasonable conversation and when making a statement of some kind the response is completely off the planet. Sometimes just a bit of conversation is genuinely needed and is missed greatly. After all, I have been talking to or listening to (more listening than talking I suppose) to this Lady for about 66 years and maybe longer.

AND THE JOURNEY CONTINUES...

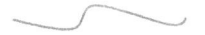

I have learned that soon we will have to forego eating out because it is very hard to please her and very often the table gets quite messy. We have enjoyed that luxury for all of our married life although for a first few years it was simply McDonalds but we thought that it was the greatest thing on the planet.

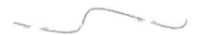

I have learned the greatness of the pain of watching the dearest person on earth not only dying mentally but now physically as well. Her condition physically seemed to have taken a hit quickly and is failing quickly. She is still beautiful but she is going downhill quickly.

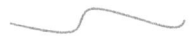

I have learned that it is very important to know when it is time to get help. The health of both patient and caregiver hangs in the balance and to be too late in getting help is not good for anyone involved. I have mentioned this before but the further we go on this journey some of the things that have already been mentioned, come back afresh again and again.

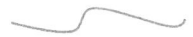

I have learned that it is very important to do the best that you can to find time for prayer and Bible study. It is really hard to do that because the patient is usually right on your heels wanting to help what you may be doing or needing you to help with something that they need or think that they need your help for. Time is such a vital thing so when it is available, grab it and use it for a good purpose. (I was just now involved in getting some very urgent work done and she came in twice to talk to me about her sister who has been dead for several years but was telling me that we needed to help her).

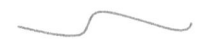

I have learned the chewing gum that she loves is the best way that I have found to keep her quiet when I am doing something that needs to be done. What is that old song about 'Chewing gum'?

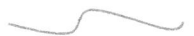

I have learned that it is impossible to know when she is really hurting and when she just thinks that she is hurting. I want her to be as comfortable as possible, but sometimes she simply hurts only in her mind and we try to distract her and she finds that she really isn't hurting at all. However, it doesn't hurt to take her to the doctor and let him run tests and see if she really has a problem.

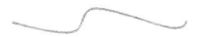

I have learned that the best remedy for a temper tantrum or a time of intense confusion is a tight and honest hug for a couple of minutes. She loves hugs especially from me and has often come to me and said, "Would you hold me?" Now that always makes me feel bad, but she has been doing that for almost 65 years. In fact, isn't that the remedy that most of us need to share?

AND THE JOURNEY CONTINUES...

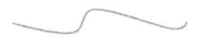

I have learned that the most painful time is when she has that flash of complete awareness of what is happening and cries and says, "I don't want to go where I am going and I don't want to leave you and the kids." Oh, the pain in my heart because I don't want her to go either but there is nothing to be done.

I have learned that the time a caregiver spends with an Alzheimer's patient without any communication from others should not be a very long time. It is really hard to go for hours, not to mention days, without anyone dropping by for just a visit and give the caregiver the opportunity to visit with someone who is aware of what is being said and is able to have a normal conversation. You may consider this to be bold but it is what I have personally learned. 5/10 minute visits can make a huge difference in a 24 hour day.

I have learned that is extremely hard to see her really struggle to do something that she has done all her life and not be able to do it. She will say, "Would you like for me to fix you something to eat?" I know that she can't, and it breaks my heart to say, "No, we'll get something later." She struggles to fold clothes and most of the time they have to be done over but I let her do it in the way that she wants to do it. She needs very much to feel needed and so I not only allow her to do things but encourage her to do them.

I have learned that nothing will replace calmness even though it is really challenging at times. Sometimes the ability to be calm seems to have become a stranger but, it is necessary to be calm and the calmness will be repaid in the same way after a few minutes.

I have learned to be very grateful that she still knows me with an occasional exception and then only for a flash of time and she laughs and recognizes me quickly. So many have asked me, "Does she still know you?" She knows me, our family, and most other people—and if she doesn't, she is an expert at faking it.

I have learned that my journey is one of its own and like no other. Others may have had similar circumstances but none have had exactly the same circumstances as mine. So, don't go telling me, "I know exactly how you feel." No, you may have lost your wife, but you didn't lose mine! You may know what it is like to lose *your* wife but you didn't lose *mine* and I didn't lose *yours*, so there is a difference.

I have learned that when my children encourage me to go to the Holiday Inn Express for a night and let them take care of My Lady, my body may be at the Holiday Inn Express but my mind is right where My Lady is and I cannot sleep for wondering about her. I do appreciate the offer, especially if they pay for it.

AND THE JOURNEY CONTINUES...

I have learned that it is highly tiring to try to watch almost every move that My Alzheimer's patient makes in order to find that something that I was going to need soon, but which she found and felt the need to hide. And, when I finally found it stashed away somewhere, she was as puzzled as me how it got to its hiding place.

I have learned that if we really had as many people living in this house as she believes we do, we would be heavily overcrowded. And those people cause me much anxiety. As I mentioned in an earlier post, "They" have become permanent residents at our house.

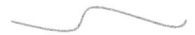

I have learned that the pain of watching My Lady being slowly taken away from me is impossible to measure. And yet, she is my greatest encourager when she assures me that everything is going to be OK. She will take me in her arms and assure me that I should not worry about her and the future. She assures me that she is not going to leave me because I couldn't make it on my own. Mercy, how can she be so strong?

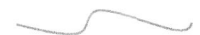

I have learned that an Alzheimer's patient becomes afraid at the slightest thing. The joking with her that I have done all of our lives now must be done very little and with great care. If she wakes up in a good spirit and seems almost normal I may get her to laugh at something silly but if the moment is not just right I must wait until another time lest the silliness is replaced with fear. Be careful with the joking.

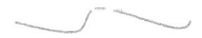

I have learned that the journey does not get easier but that I just have to catch that special moment when things seem almost normal but knowing that it is only for a moment. As quick as a flash of lightning the darkness invades again and we move on.

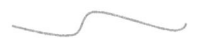

I have learned that one of my best friends is sleep because I am away from the horror of Alzheimer's for that time. But it is hard knowing that when I open my eyes the next morning, probably the first words that I hear will make no sense at all and we are plunged into the pit of Alzheimer's again.

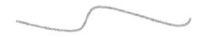

I have learned to try to be calm when outrageous statements are made that surprise and shock me. For instance, we were at the river and a barge was moving slowly along. She said, "I was on there yesterday. I flew in and landed on it." What do you do but shake your head and look away without comment.

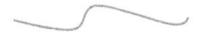

I have learned that whatever I am doing, she is going to want to help. So, I try to find something that she can help with and get her to do that. Folding clothes, helping to make the bed, washing dishes even if you have to wash them over, and other things like that will help her to feel that she is contributing.

AND THE JOURNEY CONTINUES...

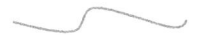

I have learned that it is OK to feel cheated when you see everyone else continuing with their lives as always before and you cannot do so. It is at that time that you really need a break for a few hours and be with someone with whom you can have a normal and pleasant conversation by going to lunch or something of that nature.

I have learned that Alzheimer's, like Satan, never stops or rests from its horrible efforts. It never says, "I have done enough damage and taken away enough from you so I will stop." It keeps slowly taking away from its prey and doesn't stop until death.

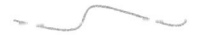

I have learned that those medical experts who tell us Alzheimer's patients do not know what they have and are not aware of what is happening to them, are very, very wrong. I wonder how many of the experts have ever lived 24/7 with an Alzheimer's patient. There is a huge difference in studying test results and in living with that patient all day, every day. I believe that there are times when My Lady is fully conscious of what is happening to her. She was lying quietly beside me and said, "You don't want to go where I am going and I am going fast." When she was rudely and abruptly told, "You have Alzheimer's" she knew exactly what that meant. There have been many occasions when she has said and done things that keenly shows that she knows exactly what is wrong with her, what her future holds to some degree, and nothing can be done to stop it. It is at those times when she is calm and quiet, and fully in control of her emotions. They are sad times but sweet times too. Don't underestimate the mental ability of an Alzheimer's patient to know what is going on in his/her world.

I have learned that no one has all the answers as to how to deal with Alzheimer's. It affects each person differently and therefore what helps with one person aggravates another. Each case must be handled with what is best for each one. That is why this message is not designed to offer advice or suggestions to do things the way that we have done them.

I have learned that it is hard to determine what confusion is and what a pure mean spirit on the part of the Alzheimer's patient is. I have thought at times that My Lady knew exactly what she was doing when she was causing so much trouble but most of the time knew that it was the disease controlling her thoughts and actions. It is really hard to deal with that kind of issue.

I have learned that it is absolutely possible to have a very, very good day and a very, very bad day on the same day because a change of feelings come that quickly. We recently had a Sunday when we attended the morning services of the church and it was a wonderful experience. However, in the afternoon she had a tremendous change of mood and by bed time I had to call our daughter for help in getting her to bed. Such a day is extremely hard to deal with.

AND THE JOURNEY CONTINUES...

I have not learned how to deal with My Alzheimer's patient's anger. Sometime she becomes very, very angry and it is very hard to know what to do or say. She has left my daughter and me both in tears as we looked into her eyes and listened to her words of intense anger. It is really a difficult problem.

I have learned that she comes almost to the place of being combative and it is then that I simply walk away and pray for wisdom to deal with this as I would with a baby. At this point she has not attempted to hit us or physically attack us but in my opinion she has come close.

I have learned that when something happens that we can share a big laugh about, it is one of the best times that we have. Sometimes she will just burst out laughing and I don't have a clue what is going on but she does and whatever it is, I love it. So I try to make those things happen as often as possible. Laughter overcomes anger and a host of other problems.

I have learned that in this highly technological age, videos should be made of family members enjoying great times together. I would give everything if I could see a video of her bustling smile and laugh, hear her laughter, see her eyes shining so brightly, and her beautiful face looking at us with hope for the future and grace that would fill me. I do not have one single video of her and it breaks my heart.

I have learned to never say 'never' when it comes to doing things that you had never thought you would do. That idea just vanishes when it comes to doing something for one so priceless and precious as the one whom you have known all of your life and have been married to for almost 64 years. One does what is best for the patient although that requires doing things that are unpleasant.

I have learned that if the Alzheimer's patient can laugh at himself/herself at times, it can be a precious time as patient and caregiver can enjoy a time of pleasant exchanges now and then. If she gets the chocolate from a Magnum ice cream bar all over her shirt and thinks it is funny, just join in the laughter and enjoy it. After all, that is why you have a washing machine isn't it?

AND THE JOURNEY CONTINUES...

I have learned that I forget all this advice that I share with you. Her mood changed this morning in the twinkling of an eye, going from someone sweet and tender to someone who was mad and mean. I am not accustomed to the moods changing so quickly. But, it won't be long 'til she will be back.

I have learned that when I look her straight in the eye, I try to remember those eyes when she was conscious of the thoughts that we exchanged before Alzheimer's. I just can't bring myself to see who she is now mentally, but to remember who she was.

I have learned that other people who know us and should expect her response to their questions and other comments to not be normal, don't respond sometimes in tender and caring way. I know that it is easy to be caught off guard but when we know the situation we just need to make a little extra effort to respond in the right way.

I have learned that LOVE is an absolutely invaluable necessity when being a caregiver for an Alzheimer's patient as well as other illnesses. It must be remembered that we are dealing with an illness which the patient has no control over. It is easy to forget that your loved one is ill and not just very difficult to get along with. Love, Love, Love, the patient and hope that it is returned—and often it is.

I have learned that if it is possible, two people need to work together in caring for an Alzheimer's patient. The hours get really, really long when you are alone. That word, 'Alone' sends awful thoughts through my head and chills through my body. It is scary.

I have learned, and this is really hard, but there have been times that I have wished that I could just go to my place of rest but I do not want to leave her for others to care for. I know that is a selfish view but at the same time it is a beautiful view.

AND THE JOURNEY CONTINUES...

I have learned that anyone who might think that staying at home and not having to go to work, but just staying with a person who is tragically ill, is the life, has not been faced with such a challenge. I would joyfully exchange what I am doing to have her well and both of us go work in a factory every day.

I have learned that it is difficult to sit and look at a person with Alzheimer's who is in good health otherwise, and to make a distinction between the person and the disease. It seems that they should be able to talk and do things as they always have but Alzheimer's has control over them and they can't. It is really, really hard.

I have learned that it is hard when you are asked, "Did God do this to me?" What do you say? I said as emphatically as I could, "NO! God did not give you this, Satan did!" She knew what I was saying and knew that it was the truth, but the question continues to haunt her at times when she knows what is happening. I will not deny that the same question has not haunted me a few times. But, I am glad that I know the correct answer.

I have learned that she still at times says some really great things. We both were in a good mood and had just laid down on the little bed in my office and I said, "Wouldn't it be good if the Lord just took both of us home right now?" "No," she said. I asked, "Don't you want to go home?" "Yes, but what about leaving the kids without us?" I said, "Well, they are 59 and 56 years old and have their own kids and grandkids. They would be just fine." "Well," she replied, "Let's just not go today."

AND THE JOURNEY CONTINUES...

I have learned that some of the very basics I have learned are how to be in tears one moment and shuddering with heartache the next. Learning to make changes so quickly presents a big challenge but keep working on it and try to make it better.

I have learned that HOPE is the anchor and the foundation that gives one a positive attitude. I know that research and medical professionals say that there is no cure for Alzheimer's and I believe that. But I have a greater and more powerful resource than that upon Whom I can fully rely. My hope is not in those people and those things but in God with whom all things are possible.

I have learned that if I sit and think of what I have lost and am losing since My Lady has Alzheimer's, I will become weaker and weaker and even my faith will be threatened. So, I try to remember the good and focus on what we can still do even as she weakens. And, even with her illness we are still winners and not losers since we have known each other from the time we were ages 7/5.

I have learned the joy of her still sitting in the audience and I can still look out and our eyes meet as she continues to say, "Go on, do a good job of preaching the gospel. It will be alright."

I have learned that sometime I am more of a baby than she is. I know that in many ways she is just a child and then I respond to her childishness as a child myself. I pray constantly that God will help me to grow up and not hurt her by being a baby myself.

I have learned that I must do things that I never dreamed that I could or would do. But, when the need comes from the most precious thing on earth to me, I can do it without hesitation and be happy to do so.

I have learned that when there is disagreement I must be the one to give in and maybe approach the subject in a different way or wait a few minutes and she will have forgotten what it was all about.

AND THE JOURNEY CONTINUES...

I have learned that it is so sad that the simple pieces of knowledge are taken from an Alzheimer's patient. That person does not know 'front from back' as in 'go to the front of the car or to the back,' They do not know 'up from down' as in 'pull your pants up or down.' So many, many, very simple things are lost to them and I want to say, "What is the matter with you?" when I tell her to go to the front of the car and she goes to the back. Then, I know what is wrong with her and it breaks my heart over and over again.

I have learned that many things have to be learned over and over again because at the pace that things are moving it is easy to forget until the same thing happens again. My older age would have nothing to do with this of course.

I have learned that even with the very best of intentions, it is difficult not to lose your temper occasionally when fierce stubbornness sets in and refuses to leave. Stubbornness is a real issue regardless of where it comes from but especially from a woman that already had an issue with it and then comes down with a horrible disease.

I have learned that sometimes it is easy to forget that the Alzheimer's patient is sick because everything seems so normal much of the time. Then the shock and surprise comes when something completely off the plate happens and for a few seconds you forget what you are dealing with.

I have learned that what I consider regular voice for me sounds like 'yelling' to her and she hates to be yelled at. We have always dealt with this because I am a loud talker. Just ask anyone who has heard me preach. So, if possible turn the volume down and it will make the patient much happier. We have shirts that say, on hers, "Don't yell at me" and on mine, "I'm not yelling."

I have learned that touching is very sensitive. I can sometimes just gently touch her ankle while trying to get her socks or hose on but to her it must be a painful attack of some kind. Both our daughter and I have been accused of hurting her when we just simply touched when she didn't want to be touched

I suppose. So, give more attention to touching and take the time to explain what you are about to do.

I have learned that she CAN'T do most of the things that she once did. I ask her to help me make the bed and sometimes she can and at other times I have to ask her to sit down and let me finish the job. It fascinates me that she CAN'T do those simple things and I MUST keep in mind that it is not possible for her to do the things that she has always done. For instance, I was encouraging her to dry off good after her shower. After I had to tell her over and over she finally wrapped the towel around her and almost yelled at me, "I don't know how." That broke my heart to pieces.

I have learned again and again that she hates the word Alzheimer's. How could she hate it if she did not know what she has as some proclaim? I would encourage everyone to be careful in your use of that word around an Alzheimer's patient because of the disturbance that it may cause in their mind.

AND THE JOURNEY CONTINUES...

I have learned that as the disease moves forward, flashes of high temper increase as well. This is when deflecting to something else or simply stopping and laying down for a little while is really needed. Often we get her to lay down on the couch, get her favorite blanket to roll up in, and she goes to sleep and rests. Sometimes I even lay down with her.

I have learned that it is a great blessing when I come to the end of my prayer she will say, "Thank you God Christ name amen." I know that some believe that a woman cannot pray in the presence of men, including her husband. I believe that the sweetest and maybe most fruitful prayers that I have ever heard have come from My Lady's lips.

I have learned to feel the pain of hurting her feelings, often by just not being in control of my temper the way I should be. I find myself saying over and over again, "She can't, She can't," before it really sinks in. The pain that comes from hurting her is almost unbearable.

I have learned to treasure the time in the evening when we can call it a night and go to sleep before I get up the next morning and pray for a short day when we can go to sleep again. This sounds confusing, but I love long nights and short days now that we are involved in this battle.

I have learned that the pain of loneliness does not disappear but grows as each day passes. Friends and family do not need to be oblivious to the existence of a loved one who needs others far more than you can ever imagine unless you have been a caregiver for an Alzheimer's patient. (Some folks seem to think that Alzheimer's is contagious like Covid and they need to stay away.) People need people to help bear this burden.

I have learned that all of the learning that I have learned must be learned over and over again. There is no such thing as thinking that I have learned something and will never have to deal with that issue again. The issue is repeated over and over again.

I have learned that Alzheimer's never gives up and will never lose its grip on someone. And, to some degree Alzheimer's has almost as much grip on the caregiver as it does its patient. It seems that both are going down together.

AND THE JOURNEY CONTINUES...

I have learned that the caregiver must learn how to better and more gently respond to angry outbursts from the Alzheimer's patient. There must not be an angry response from the caregiver to the patient but it is often very hard not to. So, back off very early to the anger and do not get into a prolonged exchange.

I have learned that it is sometimes very difficult eating in a restaurant. The noise creates disturbance and confusion in an Alzheimer's patient. It is better to have those problems at home than in public.

I have learned that as the disease progresses my heart seems to skip beats and the pain progresses as well. Prayer to God and the feeling of His loving arms is the primary source of relief. Pray often and pray deeply. I often, in my loss and pain forget to do this as I should.

I have learned that the smallest thing—a look, a whisper, a touch, and many other things—can result in a feeling of anger and or fear in the Alzheimer's patient. Please make sure to do all that you can as a caregiver to convey the right message.

I have learned that every sound is an alert for danger or some other action. The closing of a door, the ice maker, the washing machine changing cycles, unloading the dishwasher, or just a normal cracking noise of some sort does not escape her hearing and wanting to know, "What's that?"

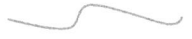

I have learned the hurt and pain that comes with watching the slow decline of the one that I love with all of my heart. It is such a miserable disease and causes so much suffering for so many people.

I have learned over and over that exhaustion is so devastating and while going through the exhaustion you may not eat properly and that compounds the problems. A caregiver must make time to rest and eat or the results can be costly.

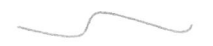

I have learned that some people cannot be as thoughtful as they should be. A lady came to us recently and stood right in our face and said, "My sister has Alzheimer's and doesn't even know who she is. She has to be fed because she forgets to eat." My Lady dropped her head and made a painful facial expression and I just wanted to take her in my arms and hold her so tightly. Please be cautious before making statements before an Alzheimer's patient.

AND THE JOURNEY CONTINUES...

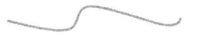

I have learned that everything in the house belongs to her and it should be put in a different place. So, get ready to look for whatever you need because it has been moved and often hidden. It gets funny as we find things that only she could have put it where we found it, but before anything is said, she firmly declares, "I didn't put that there." And, then we have a good laugh because for a flash she knows that she did.

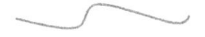

I have learned that she is part Raccoon and moves things all over the house in the most difficult place to find. Nothing is out of her reach and everything belongs to her and she can do whatever she wants to with it. So, get ready to be Sherlock Holmes if you live with an Alzheimer's patient.

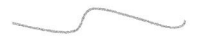

I have learned what it means to live without being able to consult with and talk to the person whom I have been married to for 64 years and 57 days and who has been my 'go-to person' for all this time. Oh, how I need her shoulder to cry on and her wisdom to help me know what to do. Ask her for help as much as you can because she might surprise you at what she remembers in a specific situation.

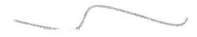

I have learned that when she is patient and kind with a sweet smile on her face, such a moment is to be cherished because it may go away for a longer period of time each time that it happens.

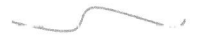

I have learned to sing more with her because it is amazing how she remembers words to a song when nearly all other memory is lost. In fact, we often sit in the swing and sing and when I forget some of the words, almost every time she can sing right on through them. This is amazing to me. Now, if all the world could be a song...

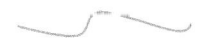

I have learned that when it is quiet and peaceful she comes up with some really good thoughts. She said yesterday, "Babies should never die, people should be kind to one another, and flowers should be everywhere, but that isn't the way that it is. But, God is still in control and everything will be alright." What beautiful thoughts. Wouldn't it be great if they came from a person who is not ill.

I have learned that the front porch swing is a wonderful place to spend as much time as possible. It is there that we sing, she seems to be at peace, we speak to and wave at the neighbors across the street or are walking in the street and she seems so relaxed and peaceful. Except when she thinks that she sees a spider and then peace and quiet have gone out the window.

I have learned that she is very particular about everything being neat and in the place that it should be. She can be given a small blanket and she will work for a long time getting the corners exactly right and if she can't get everything to match perfectly she will start over again and again.

AND THE JOURNEY CONTINUES...

I have learned that I must sacrifice my way many times when it conflicts with her way, instead of getting involved in an argument. It is good though because in a few minutes she has forgotten that there was a disagreement. It is not really all that hard to give in unless it is an issue of major importance.

I have learned to lay down with her and go back to the beginning and tell her over and over where we began our married life together. I even love to go over it myself from our beloved Michigan City, Indiana to Conway, Arkansas, and all the places between the two. And of course it makes her happy to go back to the cotton patch when we were kids together and worked in the same cotton field. The past gives an uplift it seems, and I am glad to make the trip again and again.

I have learned, to my regret, that my patience and temper is challenged greatly at times and I pray and pray that I can pull things back together without causing both of us to feel worse than we do.

I have learned that it is absolutely impossible and is a waste of time and effort to try figure out Alzheimer's. Where it comes from, how it works, etc., are questions which may never be answered. But, the results of it are plain and very painful so I am focusing on how I might best attend to the needs of both my Alzheimer's patient and myself, the caregiver.

I have learned that expecting too much of an Alzheimer's patient is painful to the caregiver. When the patient has been driven to crying out, "I can't" or "I don't know how," it is sad indeed for both the patient and caregiver. Learning to accept that the patient cannot do what we expect them to do is a much better exercise.

AND THE JOURNEY CONTINUES...

I have learned that trying to be an effective caregiver without God's help through prayer is a lost cause. That prayer closet should be the busiest place in the house. You can cry out to God in anger and frustration and He will understand. You can cry out to God for help and strength and He will give it to you.

I have learned that change comes and that it comes quickly. You often are struck almost blind by how fast the changes come. So, do your best to make as much preparation as you can for the changes that will come.

I have learned that one who is living with and caring for an Alzheimer's patient must be very careful about the things you say and the way you say them because you may live with regret for not being careful.

I have learned that pain can be deep and lasting. There is nothing that will ease the pain except Jesus, loving family and friends, prayer and Bible study, and a heart full of wonderful memories.

I have learned to attempt to the fullest of my power not to say or do things that will cause pain to the Alzheimer's patient. You know why? That patient will not remember those offenses but the caregiver will! And, guilt is a very painful thing and little cure for it.

I have learned that we are blessed when our Alzheimer's patient has a good appetite and is eager to eat. She will eat and then an hour later say, "I am starving, when are we going to eat?" And, she could eat something each time. Others whom I have heard from tell me that their patient does not want to eat at all.

I have learned that few living people understand Alzheimer's. And, I believe that there are few if any cases which are alike. I have not been able to respond to my Alzheimer's patient correctly in so many ways because I simply did not understand what she was saying or doing nor why she was responding in the way that she did.

I have learned that I need to as much as possible walk in her shoes. For instance, there were times when she could get in the car and buckle her safety belt without any reservation. The next time could not buckle nor even identify the safety belt. Then, one day I sat in the passenger seat while my son-in-law was driving and found out that her belt was much more difficult to operate than the driver's side was.

I have learned to do things that were painful mentally to both of us. I have gotten completely in the shower with her in order to give her a good shower because she simply didn't know how to do it. I have almost dragged her to the bathroom in the wee hours of the morning because she could not walk steady enough in her sleepiness to get there and take care of herself. Caregiving is not easy.

I have learned the pain of My Lady coming to me and saying, "Can I help you?" And almost every time I would be doing something that only I could do. When our daughter would be cooking she would always want to help, and some of the time she could help. However, we had to be careful of her burning herself or in some other way hurting herself in the kitchen.

I have learned that the pain is severe when the caregiver continues to give instructions and finally the patient screams, "I don't know how." This memory will live with the caregiver long after the patient has forgotten it. The failure to remember that the patient does not know how to do simple things brings regret and pain.

I have learned some well-meaning family and friends will offer advice when they don't know squat about living with an Alzheimer's patient so the caregiver must learn to use the good advice and throw out the trash. Even some who have experienced living with Alzheimer's may be wrong in the advice to your patient. No two are exactly alike so appreciate and use what is good in your case but do not feel bad to throw out what is not good for you.

I have learned that we must learn some very important words in dealing with an Alzheimer's patient. Here are some of them: Gentleness, patience, kindness, longsuffering, and there are many more of the same or near same that will bless the life of both the patient and the caregiver. Hatefulness, anger, impatience, and other spirits will break the heart of the patient and we may never see it.

I have learned to be grateful for a family whose love for their Mother, Grandmother, and Great-Grandmother is immeasurable. And, their love for a heartbroken man whose grief is also immeasurable, Father, Grandfather, and Great-Grandfather keeps him alive and moving toward that home in heaven forever.

I have learned...one time in very early hours I awoke thinking that I could hear some women talking. I got up and walked through the other part of our house and heard nothing. As I came closer to our bedroom I could hear it again and then saw that the bathroom/closet door was closed and there was no light shining under it. I opened the door quickly and turned on the light. She was standing in the closet with her face buried in clothes saying, "Help me! Someone help me please." She was in total darkness and could not find her way out of there. That one action will go with me forever. I normally woke up every time she got out of the bed, but missed this one. My heart breaks just writing about it.

I have learned that the last things that happen between husband and wife are so precious. We were lying on the bed and I knew that she was nearing the end. She had her eyes closed and several of the family members were present and we were just talking to her and loving her. Suddenly she smiled and puckered up her lips for a kiss. You cannot imagine the thrill that ran through my heart.

I have learned that one of the memories that haunts me was her having to come to me and ask, "Would you hold me a little bit?" Even when everything else may have been far away to her, the need to be held was there. Oh, how I wish that I would have been more attentive to her and all other things set aside while I held her for a little bit. Be a holder, a hugger, a kisser, and tell your loved one very often that you love him/her.

I have learned that when my Alzheimer's patient left me, my heart broke into a million pieces. She has been gone now for 238 days, but she left me two days earlier because she continued to breathe but was not aware of anything during those two days. I have learned now the awful pain that comes when Alzheimer's finally takes away its victim and you are left alone to hear the echoes of the soft and gentle breathing as the patient passes. I hate the word, "Dead." It is so cold and so permanent. If I could live for one million more days upon this earth, My Lady would never be a part of it. My Lady took one last breath upon this earth and then woke up in Paradise and will later be in heaven forever. Our earthly journey together lasted for 64 years and 96 days. She went to her rest on October 28, 2022.

I walk through the rooms and even call her name but there is nothing but silence. She will never be present with me again upon this earth and that brings to me a pain that is indescribable. So, this journey ends and a new one begins. And while the pain is almost unbearable, the joy is felt, and I await the time when I can join her and the angels to praise God forever.

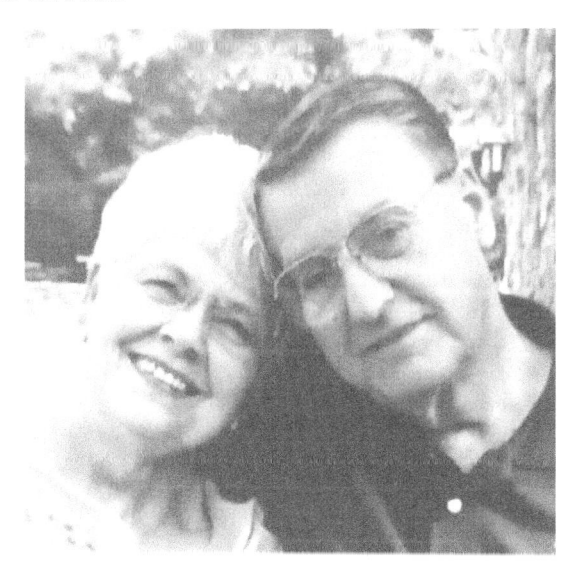

Made in the USA
Columbia, SC
19 April 2025